SURVIVALIST'S BOOK OF WISDOM

by
David Scott

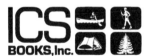

ICS BOOKS, Inc.
Merrillville, IN

Survivalist's Little Book of Wisdom

Published by: **Printed in the U.S.A.**
ICS BOOKS, Inc.
1370 E. 86th Place   Icon Illustrations by Jon Cox
Merrillville, IN 46410
800-541-7323   Cover photo: PhotoDisc

Library of Congress Cataloging-in-Publication Data

Scott, David.
    Survivalist's little book of wisdom / by David Scott.
    p.   cm. -- (Little book of wisdom series)
    ISBN 1-57034-064-1
1. Wilderness Survival.
              I. Title. II Series .
              GV2000.5.S39 1997
              613.6'9--dc21   96-38155
                                         CIP

Dedication:

To Scott Power…a survivor in the truest sense of the word.

Special Thanks to:

My family, Nicole Villanueva, Mark Bonfield,
Doc Forgey and Tom Todd.

Foreword

Throughout most of man's history, survival was not an optional skill but a way of life. Lacking the knowledge of your surroundings and not knowing how to use what was at hand meant certain death. Since then tremendous advances have been made in the outdoor industry allowing us to enjoy the wilderness more safely. The gear is better, and the techniques are more refined.

While these advances are truly remarkable, they provide many a wilderness traveler with a false sense of security. There are those who believe because they are packing a $400.00 tent and sporting a $200.00 pair of boots, nothing could possibly go wrong. There are also those who believe because they can tie 100 different knots and name a thousand different plant species, they can handle anything.

Don't misunderstand me, good gear and practical skills are without questions key to enjoying the wilderness safely, but lacking just a few basic skills of survival could cost you your life.

Survival is perhaps the most important and most neglected skill of the outdoor enthusiast. More often than not, the tragic stories we hear regarding fatalities in the backcountry happen to experienced outdoorspeople with functioning equipment. Learning the skills of survival not only helps our confidence in the wilderness, it also helps us understand our connection to and dependency on the wilderness.

No matter what your outdoor interest, survival is a skill you should not be without, and this little book is a great place to start, however like all skills survival requires practice, practice, practice. So whether you're a backcountry ranger in the mountains of Alaska, or a casual hiker in the Indiana Dunes National Lakeshore, make sure you carry in your pack the right gear, and in your mind the knowledge needed to survive.

Preface

Learning just a few tricks will greatly increase your chance of survival in the event something goes wrong. Consider this a "Cliff Notes" series on survival, a book that's trimmed the fat and delivers 357 interesting and educational trips that will help you feel more safe on your next outing.

1. Reading a good book on survival does not guarantee you will live through a survival situation.

2. Practice survival skills and experiment with them before you need to use them.
   -Karen Horney

3. Try not to eat anything unless you have water to drink with it.

4. When considering what is edible, one must loose all inhibitions i.e. do not succumb to plate fright.

5.   When a man is finally boxed and he has no choice, he begins to decorate his box.

-John Steinbeck

6.   Rain collection can also be utilized as a water source.

7.   Perspiration wastes water.

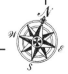

8.   Shelter is the most important element in any survival situation.

9.   Prepare yourself mentally before going on a trip by considering any possible dangers.

10. If you can't tell by touch whether or not wood is dry, touch the wood to your lips.

11. When using the previous technique, make sure there is no poison ivy or other such plants clinging to the wood.

12. Do not fall under the misconception that if animals can eat it then it must be safe for humans.

13.   The hard soil and four months of snow make the inhabitant of the northern temperate zones wiser and abler than his fellow who enjoys the fixed smile of the tropics.

-Ralph Waldo Emerson

14. If water is scarce, all travel should be done at night with a slow steady pace to keep from sweating.

15. He has not learned the lesson of life who does not everyday surmount a fear.
    -Ralph Waldo Emerson

16.   E-coli and other water-born bacteria
       incubate in about 3 days.

17.   Viruses incubate in 12 hours.

18. No passion so effectively robs the mind of all its powers of acting and reasoning as fear.

-Edmund Burke

19. The men who learn endurance, are they who call the whole world, brother.

-Charles Dickens

20.   An ounce of action is worth a ton of theory.

-Friedrich Engels

21.   Cottonwood and willow trees are very good indicators of a water source as are plants such as cattail and reeds.

22.   Building shelters in dense brush restricts your visibility.

23.   Knowing what you can not do is more
       important than knowing what you can
       do. In fact, that's good taste.
                                    -Lucille Ball

24.   Most wilderness areas are abundant
       with edible plants and animals.

25.   A good fire can be a mental comfort as
       well as a physical one.

26.   He is the best sailor who can steer within fewest points of the wind, and exact a motive power out of the greatest obstacles.

-Henry David Thoreau

27.   Anything with fur or feathers is edible.

28.   Man can acquire accomplishments or he can become an animal, whichever he wants. God makes the animals, man makes himself.

                    -G. C. Lichtenberg

29.   Always keep the space around your fire clear of flammable objects.

30. Pay close attention to fires that pop and crack. A forest fire may help you get spotted but will not improve your situation.

31. Man is always more than he can know of himself; consequently, his accomplishments, time and again, will come as a surprise to him.

    -Golo Mann

32. Softwoods (most trees with needles) burn quickly, generating a lot of heat and a lot of light, for a short period of time.

33. Softwoods do not produce long lasting fires or adequate coals for cooking.

34. Medium hardwoods such as cottonwood, poplar, aspen and willow, burn slower than softwoods.

35. Softwoods and medium hardwoods are great for starting fires, while hardwoods are great for maintaining them.

36. Hardwoods such as oak, maple or hickory burn slowly, providing low heat and low light.

37. Hardwoods produce solid, long lasting coals.

38. Fires made of hardwoods make great baking and slow roasting fires.

39. Most shelters can be quickly heated with the aid of hot rocks.

40. All insects must be cooked before eating as they may contain parasites harmful to humans.

41.   Man can climb to the highest summits,
      but he cannot dwell there long.
                    -George Bernard Shaw

42.   A hot baseball sized rock can boil a
      gallon of water in 15 minutes.

43.   Everybody talks about the weather, but
      nobody does anything about it.
                    -Mark Twain

44.   Only the unknown frightens men. But once a man has faced the unknown, that terror becomes the known.

-Antoine De Saint-Exupéry

45.   There is nothing that man fears more than the touch of the unknown. He wants to see what is reaching towards him, and to be able to recognize or at least classify it. Man always tends to avoid physical contact with anything strange.

-Elias Canetti

46. Observation, awareness and common sense are the keys to finding water.

47. Never confuse movement with action.
     -Ernest Hemingway

48. A small depression beneath your fire will help group the coals.

49. The walls of this depression or fire-pit should slope gradually, if they are too steep they will steal the heat.

50. Never travel away from your shelter without some sort of signaling device.

51. Make sure you have all your fire building materials prepared before striking a match.

52. An adventure is only an inconvenience rightly considered. An inconvenience is only an adventure wrongly considered.
     -G. K. Chesterton

53. At no time should one go 24 hours without water.

54. Water aids the body in all its functions, including thinking.

55. All reptiles and amphibians should be skinned and eviscerated before being cooked.

56. Blowing on fading embers will help fan a flame.

57.   There are two kinds of adventurers:
       those who go truly hoping to find
       adventure and those who go secretly
       hoping they won't.
                              -William Trogdon

58.   Carry a lighter.

59. Evaporation purifies water.

60. I am not an adventurer by choice but by fate.

-Vincent Van Gogh

61. Carry a metal match in your survival gear.

62. Certain plants provide a good source of water but do not expect them to taste like bottled spring water. More often than not their consistency will be much thicker than regular water.

63. If we do not find anything very pleasant, at least we shall find something new.

    -Voltaire

64.　When collecting water try to filter it first through a T-shirt or handkerchief. This will help remove any large particles that would otherwise get through.

65.　Never trust the advice of a man in difficulties.

-Aesop

66.   Always carry a survival kit in your car.

67.   In your car survival kit don't forget things like: jumper cables, spare tire, tire chains, matches, candles, sleeping bag or blanket, small amount of non-perishable food, medical kit, signaling device and extra clothing.

68. When we turn to one another for counsel we reduce the number of our enemies.

-Kahlil Gibran

69. Start with a small fire and add fuel as the flame grows.

70. Think ahead and carry some fire paste or fire ribbon.

71.   Drying food not only preserves but cuts its weight without cutting its calories.

72.   Foods are best when dried with smoke or sun.

73.   Foods can also be dried with wind of flame.

74. The main objective of drying is to rid the food of water.

75. Meat should be smoked until it is brittle.

76. When smoking meat, avoid using pine or other such resinous wood.

77. Freezing is probably the safest way to preserve meats.

78. Avoid getting the inside temperature of a snow shelter higher than 35° F. for it will raise the humidity and moisture content.

79.   Advice is what we ask for when we already know the answer but wish we didn't.

-Erica Jong

80.   A great fire starter is the paper-like bark from birch or cherry trees.

81.   Most cases of hypothermia happen between 30° and 50° F (1° and 10° C.).

82.   Do not inhale the smoke of pine or other such resinous woods as it is toxic.

83. If I were reincarnated, I'd want to come back a buzzard. Nothing hates him or envies him or wants him or needs him. He is never bothered or in danger, and he can eat anything.
   -William Faulkner

84. Avoid starting a fire directly on top of snow.

85.   A person can live for weeks without food, days without water but only a few hours without shelter in bad conditions.

86.   Union may be strength, but it is mere blind brute strength unless wisely directed.

-Samuel Butler

87. Whether you're using matches or not, fire building is an artform. Taking time to select, gather and structure firewood results in a brighter, hotter, longer-lasting fire.

88. Man is the only animal that can remain on friendly terms with the victims he intends to eat until he eats them.
-Samuel Butler

89. Pine pitch is a fantastic fire-starting aid. Pitch can be gathered on the end of a thin stick and placed between the tinder and the kindling.

90. Fire building requires four fuel types: tinder, kindling, primary wood and final wood.

91. Tinder is the starting phase of a fire
     consisting of anything dry and airy.

92. The inner bark of dead trees can be torn
     off in strips and fluffed between the
     palms providing an excellent tinder.

93. Tinder must be collected away from the
     ground to insure its dryness.

94.   Kindling may consist of dry twigs or slivers of wood ranging from the thickness of a needle to the thickness of a pencil best placed in a tipi fashion over the tinder.

95.   Primary wood will range from the thickness of your pinkey to that of your wrist.

96. Light to medium hardwoods such as cottonwood or aspen make the best primary wood.

97. Final wood is generally wood too thick to break and should only be placed on the fire when it is roaring.

98. Damp wood will work as final wood but dry is best.

99. Rocks in the wilderness provide a vast number of tools. such as sand-paper, grindstones, projectile points, knife blades, shelter heaters and water boilers.

100. Small birds can provide a delicious
meal but the amount of energy used to
obtain them is often not a beneficial
trade for the amount of nourishment
they provide.

101.   Books are good enough in their own way, but they are a mighty bloodless substitute for life.

-Robert Louis Stevenson

102.   Properly built snow shelters provide excellent insulation. Even in weather below freezing, the interior temperature will remain between 28° and 32° F. with a human inside.

103. This temperature can be increased with the aid of a candle or two.

104. Against boredom the gods themselves fight in vain.

     -Friedrich Nietzche

105. Bone can provide a keen edge when scored, split and ground or sharpened on a rough stone.

106. Fish can be caught using a line, trap or spear.

107. Look twice before you leap.
      -Charlotte Bronte

108. A properly built and placed fish trap will catch more fish with less effort than a line or spear combined.

109.   Fire needs air so you should see spaces
       between all twigs sticks and logs, yet
       all four phases of firewood should be in
       contact to help spread the flame.

110.   Every human being has, like Socrates,
       an attendant spirit; and wise are they
       who obey its signals. If it does not
       always tell us what to do, it always
       cautions us what not to do.
                              -Lydia M. Child

111. Save energy when trying to obtain wild game by trapping.

112. Specific traps are made for specific animals.

113. A properly made trap must appear as if it grew from the ground.

114. When creating snares, the snare-wire
      must be as small as possible.

115. Never leave traps set when you are done
      using them.

116. Check traps regularly. You're better off
      finding fresh game in a trap than a half
      eaten carcus.

117. If a piece of wood or a stick snaps with a sharp crack, chances are it is a decent piece of firewood.

118. Keep fire at least 5 feet from your shelter.

119. To fear the worst oft cures the worse.
    -William Shakespeare

120. For reasons concerning minimal impact
and personal safety, make an effort to
build your shelter no nearer than
200 feet from water.

121. There are moments when you feel free, moments when you have energy, moments when you have hope, but you can't rely on any of these things to see you through. Circumstance does that.

-Anita Brookner

122. Aside from plants, one of the easiest meals to obtain in the wilderness is fish.

123. When thinking of ways to collect food, choose techniques that expend the least amount of energy possible.

124. Boiling is the safest way to prepare meats and fish. The meat should be cut into identical sized cubes to promote even cooking.

125. If you are boiling meats drink the leftover broth for a full food value.

126. It always remains true that if we had been greater circumstance would have been less strong against us.
     -George Eliot

127. Make sure the shelter you build is not in the path of a possible avalanche.

128. In wilderness expect nothing--simply do the best you can.

129. Fortuitous circumstances constitute the moulds that shape the majority of human lives, and the hasty impress of an accident is too often regarded as the relentless decree of all ordaining fate.
    -Augusta Jane Evans

130. Great shelters can be constructed with no tools and a little effort.

131. Common sense is the measure of the possible; it is composed of experience and prevision; it is calculation applied to life.

-Henri-Frédéric Amiel

132. Most wild game is inedible without first being thoroughly cooked.

133. Eggs can be baked by wrapping them in green wet leaves and placing them in hot ashes for 20 minutes.

134. Man loves company, even if it is only that of a smoldering candle.
    -G. C. Lichtenberg

135. Open flames burn the food, coals cook it.

136. These are days when no one should rely unduly on his "competence." Strength lies in improvisation.
      -Walter Benjamin

137. It is best, if stranded in your car, to stay put. If you absolutely must abandon your car leave a not saying who you are, where you are headed, and the day and time you left.

138. When people are taken out of their depths they lose their heads, no matter how charming a bluff they may put up.
       -F. Scott Fitzgerald

139. A bow drill is a primitive means of creating fire by friction.

140. Courage is almost a contradiction in terms. It means a strong desire to live taking the form of a readiness to die.
    -G. K. Chesterton

141. A good experiment to test your roof is to dump two or three gallons of water over its top.

142. If you really trust your shelter building skills, sit inside the shelter while someone else dumps the water.

143. When is a crisis reached? When questions arrive that can't be answered.
-Ryszard Kapuscinski

144. Shelters will help keep a lost victim from wandering.

145. Experiment with different fire building techniques, materials and conditions before testing them in a survival situation.

146. Heat rocks in an outside fire and transfer them into the shelter with wooden tongs.

147. Make sure all hot coals are dusted or blown from the rocks.

148. Effort is only effort when it begins to hurt.

-José Ortega Y Gasset

149. Fire can be created with the aid of a magnifying glass by focusing a beam of sunlight on a pile of tinder.

150. Your living depends not only on your actions during a survival situation, but also any preventative actions you've taken before the trip.

151. Avoid building shelters with gaping holes for a doorway.

152. The entrance to a shelter should be just large enough to squeeze through.

153. Every great mistake has a halfway moment, a split second when it can be recalled and perhaps remedied.

    -Pearl S. Buck

154. Always select a brand of matches that says "strike anywhere" on the box.

155.   Fire without matches can be created in less than a half hour or less given ideal conditions and materials.

156.   Mistakes are a fact of life. It is the response to error that counts.

-Nikki Giovanni

157. Make sure you practice fire-making skills at home before depending on them in the wilderness.

158. A good shelter should have room to sit up and lay down.

159. The sap from maple and birch trees is potable.

160. When using the above suggestion, do not drink too much at one time as the sap is high in sugar and may cause cramping.

161. Experience is a good teacher, but she sends in terrific bills.
       -Minna Antrim

162. 50% of all people who become lost tend to run in a blind panic. This will only greatly worsen your situation.

163. You cannot over-hydrate.

164. Avoid overhanging rocks or dead limbs that appear as though they could fall when selecting a shelter location.

165. Also, avoid plant and animal hazards when selecting a shelter site.

166. Ever tried. Ever failed. No matter. Try again. Fail again. Fail better.
    -Samuel Beckett

167. A softball sized rock will provide two to three hours of warmth for every hour heated in the fire.

168. Heat with rocks only if there is no inside ground insulation.

169. A one gallon bucket of snow when melted will yield 1 qt. of water.

170. Melting ice provides a larger amount of water than melting snow.

171.   The man who has ceased to fear has
       ceased to care.

                                    -F. H. Bradley

172.   Water brought to a boil can be
       considered safe to drink.

173.   Comfort helps but certainly is not the
       primary objective of a shelter.

174. Perhaps catastrophe is the natural human environment, and even though we spend a good deal of energy trying to get away from it, we are programmed for survival amid catastrophe.

-Germaine Greer

175. You cannot survive if you refuse to adapt--a tree that does not bend with the wind will in time snap.

176. Over 90% of all bladed grasses are edible.

177. Doubt must be no more than vigilance, otherwise it can become dangerous.
    -G. C. Lichtenberg

178. When practicing shelter techniques, spend the night inside during different weather conditions, then ask yourself "Was I dry, was I warm, could I survive?"

179. God gives every bird his worm, but He does not throw it into the nest.

-P. D. James

180. A piece of flint or quartz struck with the back of a knife can create a spark capable of producing flame when the spark catches the tinder.

181. The above technique requires some practice and can be aided by using a piece of charred cotton cloth.

182. Hold charred cloth directly on top of flint or quartz and strike with steel to produce a spark, which catches on the cloth, and can then be placed into a tinder bundle.

183. Bad times have a scientific value. These are occasions a good learner would not miss.

-Ralph Waldo Emerson

184. No matter where you are and no matter how pure the water may appear, do your best to purify all water before drinking.

185. The "control of nature" is a phrase conceived in arrogance, born of the Neanderthal age of biology and the convenience of man.

     -Rachel Carson

186.   Man wants to live, but it is useless to hope that this desire will dictate all his actions.

-Albert Camus

187.   A reflector such as a rock or a wall of damp logs placed in a horse-shoe shape around the fire pit greatly increases the amount of heat you receive.

188. A reflector behind you also helps trap heat.

189. One should not confuse the craving for life with endorsement of it.
     -Elias Canetti

190. Nature has made up her mind that what cannot defend itself shall not be defended.
     -Ralph Waldo Emerson

191. Nature encourages no looseness,
      pardons no errors.
                    -Ralph Waldo Emerson

192. In America, nature is autocratic, saying
      "I am not arguing, I am telling you."
                    -Erik H. Erikson

193. Before taking any action in a survival situation, access the scene and determine what would best suit your needs.

194. Desperation is the raw material of drastic change. Only those who can leave behind everything they have ever believed in can hope to escape.
   -William Burroughs

195. Potable water can be obtained by using a solar still, which collects evaporation.

196. The solar still is a 3'x3' hole, holding a container, covered by a plastic sheet.

197. Try to place the solar still in an area that seems abundant in moisture if at all possible.

198. You can increase the productivity of a solar still by lining it's floor with freshly cut vegetation.

199. Another way to increase the performance of a solar still is by pouring bad water (saltwater, urine, muddy marsh water etc.) inside the hole of the still.

200. Practice any shelter technique before feeling as though you can depend on it in a survival situation.

201. Everything in the wilderness has a use or multiple uses.

202. Generally speaking, a howling wilderness does not howl; it is the imagination of the traveler that does the howling.

-Henry David

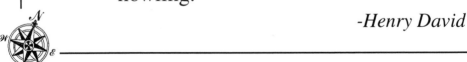

Thoreau

203.　It is not necessary to boil water for long periods of time.

204.　Man has demonstrated that he is master of everything-except his own nature.
-Henry Miller

205.　Heat is lost rapidly through conduction when laying or sitting on the ground with no form of protection underneath.

206. Nuts from oak trees or acorns have tremendous nutritional value. They should first be boiled in several changes of water, or leached in running water to remove the bitter taste.

207. Boiling meats first will tenderize the meat.

208. Broil meat as quickly as possible over hot coals. Slow roasting makes tough meat tougher.

209. If clothes become damp, maintain their protection by stuffing them with light, airy debris. This will add to overall warmth and separate wet clothing from your skin.

210. When using the previous technique, tuck your pant cuffs into your socks to keep the debris in place.

211. Stuffing clothing is called the scarecrow technique.

212. Plants such as poison ivy, or stinging nettle, make for a pretty miserable scarecrow.

213. You must be patient and not act hastily.

214. If you are in contact with the cold damp ground you will loose massive amounts of heat.

215. Within the confines of a well insulated shelter you should barely be able to hear any outside noises.

216. The hole caused by the doorway can be blocked from the inside of your shelter with the aid of a pack or extra debris.

217. You must be calm and not act irrationally.

218. Know your weaknesses.

219. Sometimes, the location in which you place your shelter can be more life threatening or saving than the shelter itself.

220. A shelter pleasing to the eye is not always pleasing to the body.

221. Don't forget a few essentials for your survival kit: signal mirror, metal match, waterproof matches or butane lighter, 50 ft. of nylon cord. knife (pocket knife with a couple tools will do) emergency blanket, water purification tablets, 7x7' sheet of 3 mil plastic, metal cup, map & compass and extra clothing.

222. You may want to augment the above kit with items such as: candles, insect repellent, energy bars, small medical kit or anything else you feel absolutely necessary.

223. Save any bones you happen to obtain as they make ideal tools.

224. Avoid toads and salamanders as a food source (shouldn't be too hard hugh?)

225. An easy, safe way to collect water is by collecting dew.

226. Use a handkerchief, T-shirt, or even a bundle of grasses to collect up to a quart of dew an hour.

227. Dew is usually safe to drink as it is a product of evaporation.

228. Dew can be contaminated by the plant from which it is being mopped or by the object with which you are mopping.

229. Dew can usually be collected very early in the morning or very late in the evening.

230. A snow shelter must be built with a vent hole placed two or three feet from the floor at a downward angle to prevent heat from escaping.

231. It is often best to collect water from a river or stream which is running swiftly and is well aerated.

232. Giardia and many other water-born parasites incubate and get you sick in about two weeks. It's more important to drink water than to purify it in a survival situation.

233. You can boil water by adding hot rocks to water in a container.

234. The container can be made from birch bark, a hollow log, leaves, or anything else that will hold water.

235.   To boil using the previous technique, remove hot rocks from the fire with wooden sticks or tongs and hold them in the water.

236.   If you are using leaves as a receptacle, do not let the hot rocks come in contact with the leaves as they will burn a hole.

237. Place eggs into water, if they sink they are edible.

238. Try to avoid eating snow (unless absolutely necessary) as a water substitute, as it takes energy to melt and can lower the body's temperature.

239. Make sure the exit of the snow cave vent hole is not so near the ground that it can be blocked by falling snow.

240. We do what we must, and call it by the best names.

-Ralph Waldo Emerson

241. Locate your shelter on the lee side of incoming weather systems.

242. Practice skills in controlled situations first, then practice under different circumstances, temperatures, and environments.

243. Boiling provides the most food value, then frying, then roasting.

244. Pound for pound, insects contain more usable protein than beef liver.

245. However much you knock at nature's door, she will never answer you in comprehensible words.
   -Ivan Turgenev

246. Avoid eating grubs with hair or bristles as some species are poisonous.

247. One of snow's greatest dangers is not its dampness but its brightness.

248. One way to improve the way in which you react to certain situations, is to control how you react to any problem, wilderness related or not.

249. Be a good animal, true to your animal instincts.

-D. H. Lawrence

250. Aside from being a fine fire starter, pine pitch serves as excellent glue. Melt into a liquid, mix in a small amount of finely powdered wood ashes, and the glue will set within a minute.

251. What distinguishes the majority of men from the few is their inability to act according to their beliefs.
-Henry Miller

252. All parts of the cattail plant are edible year round.

253. Ask yourself the proverbial "what if" questions, i.e. what if I were lost here.

254. Small shelters are beautiful shelters.

255. The wickiup (a stick and brush Tipi) is simple and quick in construction. Set three ridge poles in a tripod fashion and fill in the voids with brush and debris.

256. The wickiup is best for surviving in deserts or warmer climates. It protects well against wind and sun, but poorly against wet and cold.

257. Being physically fit helps you survive adversity.

258. Also, take into consideration the condition of your gear.

259. If you are traveling by car make sure your car is in good condition as well.

260. Never underestimate the strength and adaptability of the human body, especially when fighting for life and when supported by a positive mental attitude.

261. Loose inhibitions and don't be afraid of looking foolish.

262. Physical strength is helpful but not a determining factor.

263. Mental strength is crucial and, in most cases, the determining factor.

264. Increase a shelters warmth by covering the floor with a thick layer of pine boughs or other debris.

265. Heat ma'am! It was so dreadful here that I found there was nothing left for it but to take off my flesh and sit in my bones.

-Sydney Smith

266. If you can't stay dry while building a snow shelter, or can't get dry after it has been built, don't build a snow shelter.

267. Fear can cause a positive reaction, or a negative distraction.

268. In the world there is nothing more submissive and weak than water. Yet for attacking that which is hard and strong nothing can surpass it.

-Lao-Tzu

269. The weak are more likely to make the strong weak than the strong are likely to make the weak strong.

    -Marlene Dietrich

270. Talk to yourself out loud.

271. Half of all red berries in the U.S. are poisonous.

272. You can die in three days without water while diarrhea will normally not kill you.

273. If you get diarrhea, increase your water intake.

274. You see things; and you say "Why?" But I dream things that never were; and say "Why not?"

    -George Bernard Shaw

275. Finely dicing and steeping a small handful of pine needles in hot water provides a tea with a valuable source of Vitamin C.

276. Don't agonize. Organize.
    -Florence R. Kennedy

277. Wild fish should never be eaten raw.

278. You can't always have what you want, but you can have what you need.

279. Carrying a water purification system on a wilderness trip is as important as carrying matches. Commercial purification products on the market are all approved by the EPA.

280. Try to make the ceiling of your snow shelter as smooth as possible to decrease dripping.

281. A thin layer of leaves and grass laying on some sticks does not a roof make.

282. The debris shelter roof should be as thick as your arm is long.

283. Action helps delete the mind of negative thought.

284. When you realize you've become lost, sit down and back track mentally before trying to back track physically.

285. Trust thyself: every heart vibrates to that iron string.

    -Ralph Waldo Emerson

286. High and dry is generally a good rule, but always use common sense when building a shelter.

287. Hilltops are prone to high winds and lightning.

288. A good shelter in a bad location is a bad shelter.

289. Hindsight is always twenty-twenty.
      -Billy Wilder

290. Insulation is the key to warmth.

291. The trouble with Reason is that is
      becomes meaningless at the exact point
      where it refuses to act.
      -Bernard Devoto

292. Even when casually hiking and no problem is at hand, pay attention to things like possible fire and shelter materials along with signs of nearby animals or water supplies.

293. There is always a period of curious fear between the first sweet-smelling breeze and the time when the rain comes cracking down.

-Con Delillo

294.   The aims of life are the best defense
       against death.

       -Primo Levi

295.   Equipment should be based on three
       things: personal, geographical, and
       seasonal.

296.   When building a shelter remember, the
       smaller it is the less heat must be
       generated to keep it warm.

297. Build something near your shelter that will attract attention from the air or the ground.

298. A sharp edge can be made by striking a smooth egg shaped rock with another harder rock using a downward circular motion. Forming a flake that should be fairly sharp around the edges.

299. Do not concern yourself with making stone tools that appear to be taken from the shelf in a museum-all you need is a keen working edge.

300. Most victims lost in the wilderness are found within three days.

301. Wilderness survival is very similar to a game of chess. The game is 90% mental: you must access the entire scene, you must anticipate, you must adapt, you must overcome and you must advance.

302. Wash maggots thoroughly before boiling or cooking.

303. A simple fish hook can be made from a small stick no thicker than a pencil. It should be 2 inches long and sharp at both ends. One end of this "straight hook" should be heavier so it hangs parallel to the line rather than perpendicular making it more easily swallowed by the fish.

304. To keep a fire burning all night, use slightly greener wood or punkey wood on top of a good coal base.

305. Don't jump on wood or slam it against a tree in order to break it as these are both rather risky endeavors. Burn it in half or place it in the notch of a tree and lever it in half.

306. Try to build your shelter near an abundance of materials such as a good supply of shelter building material, firewood and water.

307. Don't build in a bad location to compliment these three things, but make an effort to have such materials close at hand.

308. Man can live for 3 to 4 weeks without eating any food.

309. Water should be stored in your stomach not in your water bottle.

310. Of all survival elements, food is the least important.

311. Be it a survival situation or not, hydration is immensely important in any wilderness situation.

312. Fear always springs from ignorance.
     -Ralph Waldo Emerson

313. If you are planning a large expedition, a course in wilderness medicine or at least a course in first-aid would be worth taking.

314. Do your best to learn some of the basics if you can't take such a course.

315. Experience is the name everyone gives his mistakes.
    -Elbert Hubbard

316. Keep your pee clear, not yellow.

317. Light colored urine means you are properly hydrated.

318. Always enter the wilderness humbly.

319. I'd rather have them say "There he goes" than "Here he lies."
    -Anonymous

320. Any wood that is in contact with the ground should be considered wet, yet it may still burn.

321. An utterly fearless man is a far more dangerous comrade than a coward.
     -Herman Melville

322. When using fire as a signal be careful not to worsen your situation by starting a forest fire.

323. The greatest accomplishment is not in never falling, but in rising again after you fall.

-Vince Lombardi

324. Never give up.

325. Never challenge the wilderness.

326. The best way out is always through.
      -Robert Frost

327. Sometimes, the best way out is *around.*
      -David Scott

328. If you are idle, be not solitary; if you
      are solitary, be not idle.
      -Samuel Johnson

329. Aside from providing a means by which to cook, fire also provides warmth, water purification, and may act as a signaling device.

330. The proverb warns that "You should not bite the hand that feeds you." But maybe you should, if it prevents you from feeding yourself.

-Thomas Szasz

331.   Be thine own palace, or the world's thy jail.

-John Donne

332.   Yet is every man his own greatest enemy, and as it were his own executioner.

-Sir Thomas Browne

333. When the beginnings of self-destruction enter the heart it seems no bigger than a grain of sand.

-John Cheever

334. Know your limits.

335. Push them from time to time.

336. One thorn of experience is worth a whole wilderness of warning.
-James Russell Lowell

337. Shelters built in dense covering take longer to dry.

338.   Survival situations can usually be broken down in three different phases: pre-accident phase, accident phase, and the recognition phase.

339.   Sometimes these phases are obvious such as a plane crash, and sometimes they are more subtle such as becoming lost.

340. The pre-accident phase often happens before you even leave the house.

341. The pre-accident phase is most often the result of improper planning and preparation.

342. Forgetting to bring certain items, not being in proper physical condition, lacking knowledge of your hiking or camping area are some classic examples of a pre-accident phase.

343. The accident phase takes place the moment you become lost whether you know it or not.

344. Each step you take after the moment you've become lost accelerates the accident phase.

345. The most crucial phase in a survival situation is the recognition phase.

346. The recognition phase happens the moment you realize something is wrong.

347. How you react during the recognition phase determines whether you live or die.

348. A person will either take action or become distraut or frozen with fear.

349. Many emotions enter the stage during the recognition phase: fear, anger, embarrassment, panic, distraction and depression.

350. These emotions can be used for or against you.

351. Probably the best thing you can do at the recognition phase is to sit down and think.

352. We'll never know the worth of water till the well go dry.
     -Scottish Proverb

353. Shelters built with southern exposure provide the longest lasting heat and light.

354. Often in winter the end of the day is like the final metaphor in a poem celebrating death: there is no way out.
    -Agustin Gomes-Arcos

355. Avoid unnecessary risks.

The Little Books of Wisdom Series

Parent's Little Book of Wisdom
by Tilton / Gray ISBN 1-57034-039-0A

Writer's Little Book of Wisdom
by John Long ISBN 1-57034-037-4A

Bachelor's Little Book of Wisdom
by David Scott ISBN 1-57034-038-2A

Traveler's Little Book of Wisdom
by Forgey, M.D. / Scott ISBN 1-57034-036-6A

Canoeist's Little Book of Wisdom
by Cliff Jacobson ISBN 1-57034-040-4A

Teacher's Little Book of Wisdom
by Bob Algozzine ISBN 1-57034-017-XA

Doctor's Little Book of Wisdom
by William W. Forgey M.D. ISBN 1-57034-016-1A

Camping's Little Book of Wisdom
by David Scott ISBN 0-934802-96-3A

Handyman's Little Book of Wisdom
by Bob Algozzine ISBN 1-57034-046-3A

Dieter's Little Book of Wisdom
by William W. Forgey M.D. ISBN 1-57034-047-1A

Musician's Little Book of Wisdom
by Scott Power ISBN 1-57034-048-XA

* Salesman's Little Book of Wisdom
by Scott Power ISBN 1-57034-061-7A

* Hiker's Little Book of Wisdom
by David Scott ISBN 1-57034-062-5A

* Golfer's Little Book of Wisdom
by Sean Doolin ISBN 1-57034-063-3A

* Survivalist's Little Book of Wisdom
by David Scott ISBN 1-57034-064-1A

*The LITTLE Gift Books That
Will be a BIG Hit For All
Your Gift Giving*

**For a Free Catalog
Call Toll Free in U.S.
800-541-7323 or 219-769-0585
Only $5.95 to *$6.95 Each**